Clogged, Narrowed and Barely Pumping

Everything You Need to Know About Coronary Artery Disease

Clogged, Narrowed and Barely Pumping

Everything You Need to Know About Coronary Artery Disease

By: Dr. Courtney Hamilton, Pharm.D., BCPS

Categories: Health and Self-help

Table of Contents

Preface

According to the World Health Organization, the leading cause of death in the world is cardiovascular disease followed by diabetes and hypertension.[1] In the United States, the Centers for Disease Control has noted that diseases affecting the heart have the greatest burden of death, taking the lives of over 600,000 people a year, most of those deaths being male.[2] The incidence of death has greatly declined over the years – secondary to improved prevention screening, proactive treatments and modifying appropriate risk factors. The only way for this curve to continue to decline is if we continue to be proactive in diagnosing and treatment.

Purpose

The focus of this book is to help you gain basic knowledge and power in the understanding of what coronary artery disease is, how it's managed, and what you can do about it. The goal of this book is to provide you with tips for you how can begin to gain control and manage coronary artery disease.

Being diagnosed with coronary heart disease or being told that you are at high risk is not the end of the world. Studies have shown that coronary heart disease can be reversed. How you ask? I hope to convey that throughout this book; but the key is to obtain knowledge about the disease state and to make some simple changes in: what you eat; exercising; and creating healthy habits. Trust me, you can improve and put a halt to the progression of this and quite possibly reverse some of the damage. I hope you find this to be a beneficial tool in your journey against heart disease.

■■■

What is Heart Disease?

The question still remains, who is this big bad guy? We often use the term heart disease to describe several types of diseases of the heart. The most common types of heart disease are coronary artery disease, stroke, angina pectoris, myocardial infarction, silent myocardial ischemia and peripheral arterial disease. The focus of this book is coronary artery disease (CAD). CAD refers to the narrowing and the hardening of blood vessels caused by atherosclerosis.

"Stop! Wait? I'm so confused. Where does it come from? What does it look like? Why is it here?"

You must be asking yourself. After all, those are all questions I asked myself.

What is atherosclerosis?

Atherosclerosis is the buildup of plaque in narrowing arteries. Plaque is made of fat, cholesterol and other substances found in the blood. The buildup of plaque can lead to blood clots from the colligating of blood that cannot adequately pass through the arteries. As a consequence, you may develop angina (chest pain), or a non-ST elevation myocardial infarction (NSTEMI) also known as advanced cholesterol plaque or a ST elevation myocardial infarction (STEMI). The difference between each of these stages is as follows: NSTEMI is when a portion of the artery is blocked causing reduced blood flow; STEMI is when the artery is completely blocked and blood cannot get through to oxygenate the rest of your body.

Where does atherosclerosis come from?

Simply put, atherosclerosis begins as plaque or buildup of fatty streaks floating in your arteries. These fatty streaks are made up of cholesterol, fat, and blood cells. They develop a hardened fibrous cap over it, decreasing the flow of blood and the amount of oxygen reaching the heart. It should be noted

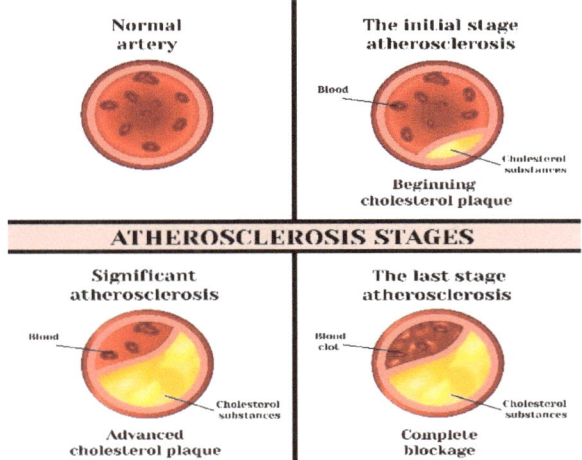

that atherosclerosis can be found throughout the body in the heart, brain, and other areas. After the development of atherosclerosis, insults such as hypertension, smoking and high blood pressure can cause injury to the endothelial lining (inner most lining of the hearts artery), releasing the contents of the plaque into the blood stream.

What does atherosclerosis look like?

Imagine the fat that you see on steak or chicken, lumped in a corner of a narrow passage way.

Why is atherosclerosis in my arteries?

Atherosclerosis is usually secondary to hereditary factors and/or our way of life. For instance, a sluggish lifestyle with little physical activity and a diet high in fat.

Effects of Coronary Artery Disease

CAD can lead to several complications such as: heart attacks, heart failure, stroke, peripheral arterial disease, aneurysm, and even sudden cardiac arrest. The most common complication is chest pain. If CAD goes uncontrolled for an extended period of time your arteries will become clogged, narrow and will have a harder time completing its daily functions like pumping blood throughout your body.

Managing Coronary Artery Disease

Diagnosing

The type of treatment your doctor may prescribe for you will be dependent on if you are at risk of developing CAD or if you have had a recent arteriosclerotic cardiovascular disease event (ASCVD); such as a heart attack or peripheral arterial disease. A formal diagnosis is assessed through these categories:

1. LDL level
2. Age
3. Diabetes
4. Previous arteriosclerotic cardiovascular disease event (ASCVD)
5. Calculated ASCD 10- year risk

Based on these factors your provider will determine how intense your treatment needs to be: low, moderate, or high intensity.

Patients at the highest risk will usually fall into 1 of 4 categories listed below per the ACC/AHA guidelines:[3]

1. Previous ASCVD event
2. LDL level greater than 190mg/dL
3. Age of 40-75, Diabetes + an LDL level 70-140mg/dL
4. Age of 40-75, an LDL level of 70-140mg/dL and an estimated ASCVD Risk of greater than 7.5%

Preventive Treatment

The type of medical treatment your doctor may prescribe for you will be based on if you have already had an NSTEMI or STEMI or if he/she is trying to prevent an occurrence. Prevention can be managed by medical intervention, natural intervention, or invasive intervention – completed by a specialized cardiovascular surgeon – or a combination of the three. Medically, your doctor can prescribe a medication from one of several drug classes: HMG-Coa reductase inhibitors, bile acid sequestrants, fish oils, ezetimbe, nicotinc acids, fibrates, and PCSK-9 inhibitors, in addition to a baby aspirin a day. To determine which agent you should use your provider will review your detailed lipid panel assessing low density lipoproteins (LDL), high density lipoproteins (HDL), and triglycerides (TG). Your provider will also assess your other diseases and medications to determine which agent will provide an optimal lipid response.

Aside from medications, the most important thing you can do to take control of your heart and arteries is to preform natural interventions – such as, management of your diet, stress and exercising regularly. More often than not, heart disease is your bodies response to another battle you have been fighting internally. The following are modifiable risk factors that will decrease your chance of developing CAD:

- Obesity
- Smoking
- Diet
- Physical inactivity
- Dyslipidemia
- Hypertension
- Diabetes mellitus

Explanation
- Obesity/Physical Inactivity – Indirectly by directly affecting several other major risk factors like high cholesterol, diabetes, and high blood pressure.
- Smoking – *Everyone is always talking about how smoking is bad for you but no one explains why.*
  In short, the chemicals released from your – cigar, cigarette, black and mild – Increase the formation of atherosclerosis by increasing blood pressure and cholesterol while reducing the amount of oxygen your blood carries throughout the body. [4,5]
- Dyslipidemia/hyperlipidemia – Directly causes congested arteries through the formation of plaque.
- Hypertension – Increases the tension/pressure in your arteries causing damage to the artery wall.
- Diabetes mellitus – Reduces your body's production of nitric oxide which causes a decrease in blood flow and makes the arteries "stickier" and easier for the fat and cholesterol to bind to.

- <u>Diet</u> – Diets high in fat have been found to contribute to the development of hyperlipidemia, hypertension, and diabetes.

But why?

Well, because everything in your body is connected. No one system can function without the other being at its best. The best way to combat CAD is to tackle each of these risk factors.

Treatment for active disease

Things get a little tricky for those who have been diagnosed as having a heart attack or any other atherosclerotic event. Treatment for those individuals will require a more detailed medication regimen and will follow the ABC rules:

Aspirin
Blood Pressure
Cholesterol
Diabetes
Exercise and Diet

Treating CAD is tricky because there are a few components outside of cholesterol which require you maintain other co-morbidities or risk factors. These patients will require an antiplatelet – like aspirin, to prevent them from passing blood clots through their arteries. Patients at risk or who have developed atherosclerosis should refrain from smoking; maintain a healthy blood pressure and blood sugar. This can be done through medication or diet and exercise, often times through a combination of these suggestions.

What kind of medications do they use?

Cholesterol medications:

HMG-Coa Reductase Inhibitors: Also known as a "statins". They mainstay of treatment according to the American College of Cardiology and the American Heart Association (ACC/AHA); due to the overwhelming amount of literature and research supporting its use. This class of medication is most commonly associated with muscle pain and fatigue. However, intolerance or muscle pain to one "statin" does not exclude you from utilizing a different medication from this class.
Notes for this medication - Works best when taken at night before you go to bed because your body produces most of its cholesterol in your sleep.
Medications in this class - Pravastatin®, Simvastatin®, Atorvastatin®, Rosuvastatin®, Pitavastatin®, and Lovastatin®.

Bile Acid Sequestrants – This medication should not be taken by patients with high levels of TG, as a common side effect is hypertriglyceridemia, along with upset stomach and constipation.
Notes for this medication – Interacts with other medications so it should be taken 2 hours before other medications or 4 hours after.

Medications in this class – Cholestyramine®, Colestipol®, Colesevelam®

Nicotinic Acids – The most common seen side effect with this medication is flushing, high blood sugar and elevated levels of uric acid. Patients with history of liver disease and gout should not take this product.
Notes for this medication – Flushing can be minimized by taking an aspirin 30 minutes prior to dose and taking at bedtime.
Medications in this class – Niacin, Slo–niacin (may also reduce flushing)

Fish Oil – When combined with diet changes reduces TG and increases good cholesterol but raises LDL slightly.
Medications in this class – Fish oil, Lovaza

Ezetimibe – Reduces both LDL and TG levels.
Notes for this medication – Headache and rash are common side effects.
Medications in this class - Zetia®

Fibrates – Reduces triglycerides with the risk of increasing LDL slightly.
Notes for this medication – Most notable adverse effects are gallstones, and elevated liver enzymes.
Medications in this class – Fenofibrate and Gemfibrozil

Commonly used Blood Pressure Medications:

<u>Ace Inhibitors</u> – Most commonly seen side effect with this class is a dry hacking cough. In addition to blood pressure control they help arteries/heart get oxygen.
Medications in this class- Lisinopril, Enalapril, Fosinopril
<u>Beta-Blockers</u> – Common adverse effects is lowered heart rate. In addition to blood pressure control they help arteries/heart get oxygen
Medications in this class – Metoprolol tartrate, Metoprolol succinate, Carvedilol, Bisoprolol, Atenolol

So, my doctor told me if I don't take my medications and work out I am going to die…

There are several methods for convincing patients to comply with their therapy plans, from "do as I have instructed" to scare tactics. But from my experience neither of those works. Patients who benefit the most are those who are actively included in their health care plan. From this step forward we are a team. You tell me…

Why did you pick up this book? Why do you care about heart disease? What were you hoping to accomplish?

The most common reasons I have heard:

- I want to be live longer for my significant other, children, grandchildren, or myself

- I want to live a more active lifestyle

- I hate the idea of needing surgery

- I don't want to be dependent on anyone

- What will happen to my family if something happens to me

- How will my family feel if something happens to me

- What would happen to my dogs/cats if I died

- I don't want to take so many pills everyday

I can promise you only one thing. If you are dedicated to your health, you will see changes. I can tell you about the complications of heart disease, but unless you are dedicated to making lifestyle changes you will not see improvement in your risk of developing heart disease.

What is in this for me?

So, now you're thinking *"alright, I'm going to make some changes, but what else do I get from this?"*

You will become empowered! Sure, it will take time, changes will not happen overnight but this is a challenge… And we like challenges! Now that you are dedicated to making changes, you will feel good! Your health will improve and all that snoring your significant other complains about? *Decreased!* And now you are sleeping better, you have more energy and more brain power! Guess what ladies? You have healthier skin and brighter eyes. Did I mention how empowered you will feel for taking over and taking control of your body and health? We only have one body so we must take care of it.

Help!

My doctor has given me a whole medicine cabinet full of DRUGS. I am OVER being drugged.

I am a pharmacist by trade and usually my patients are under the impression that I simply want to "drug them up" and send them on their way. Believe it or not, I would prefer not to. Diet and exercise can do more wonders for your body than the majority of the drugs on the market. Medications are a great way to augment and help your body make the changes it needs to—on a molecular level. Keeping a healthy weight, maintaining your diet and exercising will go much further and you will be able live a more energetic and active lifestyle.

You don't need a fancy gym membership to get in shape. You can work out in the privacy of your own home or in your neighborhood. Whether you walk/run around your neighborhood and create your own workout session with jumping jacks and crunches or you decide to use a YouTube walking video for ideas. House needs to be cleaned? Turn on some music and pull out that vacuum. Going to the grocery store or shopping at the mall? Either way put on your power moves and pick up those knees. The recommended goal is 150 minutes a week of uninterrupted cardio or 30 minutes 5 days a week. Power walking, jogging, or even cycling, they all work. Everything you do counts towards your new and improved lifestyle, which will improve your blood pressure, blood glucose and eventually your atherosclerosis.

So, again I say, know your risk. Between out of pocket costs and insurance you pay the doctor a lot of money for his/(er) knowledge, take advantage of that. Have a conversation with your provider and ask how at risk am I? What does my blood work look like and what should it look like. Never be ashamed to say "I don't understand" or "please explain this to me?" Ask your doctor what your current lab values look like and what your goal should be and then create a reasonable timeline for reaching that goal.

Write down your doctor's goals and then make your own manageable goals to work towards those set by your provider. Make a plan and progressively execute them. The key is to stay consistent in your efforts. You CAN DO IT! I believe this and you should too!

Crash Course

Here is a quick guide to review the definition of key terms you should know.

1. Cholesterol
    a. Definitions
        i. Low density lipoprotein (LDL) – Also known, as "bad" cholesterol because it helps cholesterol get around and form plaque that sticks to arteries. In good levels your body uses this to build hormones and cells.

ii. High density lipoprotein (HDL) – Known as the good cholesterol because when maintained appropriately it helps remove LDL from the arteries and your body uses this to build hormones and cells.

iii. Triglycerides (TG) – This is a fat found in your blood, that when maintained in normal levels provides the necessary energy for cellular function.

b. Why we measure cholesterol levels
   i. To help better asses if a patient is at risk for high cholesterol and indirectly to measure risk of developing heart disease.

c. How we measure cholesterol
   i. Measured through a blood sample

d. What a typical goal looks like
   i. Current ACC/AHA guidelines have stated that there is no benefit to reaching target goals for these particles. A patient/provider should strive to maintain a reduced risk of developing CAD after diagnosis. [3]
   ii. Current National Lipid Association (NLA) guidelines have stated the following as being desired goals.[3]
      1. LDL
         a. Less than 100 mg/dL
      2. HDL
         a. Men: Greater than 40 mg/dL

                    b. Women: Greater than 50mg/dL
                3. Triglycerides
                    a. Less than 150 mg/dL

2. Blood Pressure
    a. Definitions
        i. Blood Pressure – Each time your heart beats, it is pumping blood throughout your body to provide it with the oxygen, energy, and nutrients it needs. The force at which it pushes your blood through its arteries is how we determine its "pressure".
        ii. Systolic (top number) – Determines the pressure in your arteries when your heart muscle contracts.
        iii. Diastolic (bottom number) – Determines the pressure in your arteries when it is resting between beats.

    b. Why we measure blood pressure
        i. To help determine if a patient has high blood pressure, given that most patients do not usually present with symptoms of high blood pressure.

    c. How we measure blood pressure
        i. Measured by using either an automatic or manual blood pressure cuff.
        ii. Rest 5 minutes before assessing.
        iii. Do not smoke or have coffee 30 minutes before assessing.

    d. What a typical goal looks like

     i. Current Joint National Committee Guidelines recommend: [6]
        1. People greater than 60 years of age without diabetes or chronic kidney disease: less than 150/90 mmHg
        2. People 18-59 years of age without co-morbidities: less than 140/90 mmHg
        3. People 18-59 years of age with diabetes or co-morbidities: less than 140/90 mmHg

3. Glucose
   a. Definitions
     i. Fasting – May also be referred to as pre-prandial or before meals. The state in which your body has went at least 8 hours without food.
     ii. Fed – May be referred to as post-prandial or after meals. The state your body is in after eating.
     iii. A1C – Also known as, hemoglobin A1C is a test completed to determine your average blood glucose level over a 3-month period.

   b. Why we measure blood glucose
     i. To help better identify blood sugars that is too high or too low. To asses if medications are effective.

   c. How we measure for diagnosis
     i. Measured in two manners both of which are blood tests.
        1. A1C test – blood sample taken from a lab.
        2. 2-Hour glucose tolerance test (GTT) – The individual drinks a 75-gram glucose drink,

followed by a blood sample drawn 2 hours after. This test is usually completed after a fasting sample.

d. What a usual blood glucose goal is: [7]
    i. Fasting: 80-130 mg/dL
    ii. Fed: Less than 180 mg/dL
        1. This level is best taken at least 1-2 hours after the beginning of a meal
    iii. A1C: Less than 7%

Disease

- What is my diagnosis?
- Will I need surgery?
- How many blockages do I have in my arteries? How severe are the blockages?
- Am I at risk for having a heart attack?
- What additional tests may I need?
- How often will I need to come in for check-ups?
- What are your goals for me?
- Do I have any additional co-morbidities that may benefit from management?
- What are some signs that I need to go to a hospital or seek treatment right away?

Medications

- What are my treatment options? What are the benefits of each option? What are the side effects?
- How should I take them?
- How long do I have to take these medications?
- Will the medicine(s) you prescribed interact with the medicine(s) I currently take?
- Is this a cure or will it just make me feel better?

How do I get organized?

I *am so glad you asked! Keep a diary. Taking it old school.*

Keep a diary of your blood sugar, blood pressure, weight, and/or whatever else you think will help you stay organized and accountable for your changes. For the first couple of weeks keep it somewhere obvious, on your desk, or your refrigerator. I believe one of the best ways you can help your provider help you is by keeping a log so that (s)he may see if there is pattern to what causes your blood pressure or blood sugar spikes/falls. Check out Appendix C. I have created some charts to help jump start you on the right page.

■■

I like to consider myself a foodie, I genuinely love to eat. So, I have a hard time telling you "don't eat this and definitely don't eat that!" But I am a firm believer

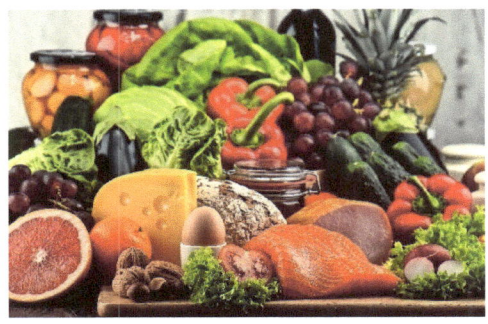

in ***knowing your limits*** and eating in moderation. If you are anything like me, you are a *see-food-eater*. I think it's the aroma I love so much. If it smells good, it's mine. But because I know this very important fact about myself I practice self-control.

I do this through 5 simple rules:
1. Know the correct portion sizes and what is in your meal
2. More veggies, less carbs
3. Drink 6-8 glasses of water!!!
4. Two meatless meals a week
5. Low-fat vs regular fat

Studies have showed that those who practice a diet high in vegetables and fruits, much like the Mediterranean diet have reduced their risk of developing cardiovascular disease.[8]

With that in mind your diet should consist of:
1. Good fats (salmon and avocado)

2. Fiber (lentil beans, and pears)
3. Whole grains (brown rice and oatmeal)

A well—balanced meal should look like so: ½ your plate is veggies! The other half is divided between your meat and your starch.

Things you should avoid:
1. Red meats
2. Saturated fats
3. High fructose corn syrup
4. Sugary foods and drinks (some juices included)

What should my pantry look like?

There are some items that should always be readily available in your kitchen. Also, as a rule of thumb stick close to the walls of the grocery store, when grocery shopping. Usually, the healthiest items are there, because they need refrigerators to keep them fresh. Meanwhile, the packaged goods that can sit around for months are located in the center aisles. This however, does not mean to shop in the freezer section for frozen foods either.

I digress, below are things we should always keep on hand (keep in mind to avoid these items if you have any known allergies):

1. Snacks
   a. Almonds
   b. Strawberries
   c. Blueberries
   d. Pineapple
   e. Pears
   f. Red Peppers
   g. Yellow Peppers
   h. Celery
   i. Humus

2. Meals
   a. Avocado
   b. Spinach
   c. Oatmeal
   d. Tomatoes
   e. Eggs (boiling is your friend)
   f. Onions
   g. Ground turkey meat

We have even shared a few recipes to help you get a jump start on a proper diet.

■■■

Recipe Kick Starter

I.   Breakfast
      a.   Avocado Toast
      b.   Strawberry Passion Parfait

II.   Lunch
      a.   Chicken chili
      b.   Baked Avocado

III.   Dinner
      a.   Avo-shrimp-ilicious Salad
      b.   Cauliflower fried rice

IV.   Dessert
      a.   Pineapple-OO-La-La

Breakfast

Avocado Toast

Total Time: 10 minutes
Prep time: 7 minutes
Cook time: 3 minutes

Yield: 2 servings

Ingredients:
- 4 slices of bread
- 10 cherry tomatoes slice long ways
- 2 avocados (peeled and sliced long ways)
- 8 dashes of pepper

Instructions:
- Use a toaster or toaster oven to toast the 4 slices of bread.
- Once the toast is complete apply slices of avocado on top
- Add 2 dashes of pepper to each slice of bread.
- Top with 5 slices of cherry tomatoes.

Strawberry Passion Parfait

Total Time: 5 minutes
Prep time: 5 minutes
Cook time: 0 minutes

Yield: 2 servings

Ingredients:
- 1 cup of strawberries sliced long ways
- ½ cup blueberries
- 1 cup of yogurt (preferred stonybrook)
- ½ cup Granola crunch

Instructions:
- In a bowl/cup mix up blueberries and strawberries
- In a separate bowl/ cup apply 1 layer of fruit mix followed by a layer of yogurt and repeat until bowl/cup is full then top with granola

Lunch
Western White Bean Chicken Chili

Total Time: 105 minutes
Prep time: 15 minutes
Cook time: 90 minutes

Yield: 4 servings

Ingredients:
- 4 chicken breast sliced and cubed
- 1 can white navy beans
- 1 can white kidney beans
- 4 stalks of celery (sliced thin)
- 1 yellow onion sliced and diced
- 1 cup of greens onions (sliced thin)
- 1 can of Mexican (fiesta) corn drained and rinsed
- 2 cans of chicken broth
- 3 tablespoons of cayenne pepper
- 3 tablespoons of pepper
- 1 tablespoons of cumin
- ½ packet of taco seasoning
- 4 tablespoons of onion powder
- 6 tablespoons of garlic powder
- 5 tablespoons of chili powder

Instructions:

- Once preparation of all vegetables is complete compile all ingredients into Dutch oven or crock pot (Crock pot cook time should be extended to at least 4-6 hours)
- Seasoning should be applied throughout the simmering of the meal. Add additional spices as necessary. (Avoid salts!)

Twice Baked Avocado

<u>Total Time</u>: 10 minutes
Prep time: 2 minutes
Cook time: 8 minutes

<u>Yield</u>: 4 servings

<u>Ingredients</u>:
- 2 Avocados cut in ½ and pitted
- 1/3 cup of shredded low fat cheese (I prefer cheddar)
- 4 dashes of pepper
- 4 dashes of cumin
- ¼ cup of yellow onions sliced and diced
- 4 cherry tomatoes sliced and diced

<u>Instructions</u>:
- Mix onions, tomatoes, and cumin and scoop into the pit of the avocado
- Apply 2 dashes of pepper to each avocado half
- Sprinkle cheese across the top
- Broil in oven for 6-8 minutes

*monitor closely—broiling food cooks much faster than baking and may result in burning.

Dinner

Avo-Shrimp-A-Licous Salad
Total Time: 20 minutes
Prep time: 10 minutes
Cook time: 10 minutes

Yield: 2 servings

Ingredients:
- 1 cup of frozen shrimp defrosted (deveined, tail-off)
- ½ bag of fresh spinach
- 3 dashes of garlic and herb seasoning (Mrs. Dash, my preferred brand)
- 3 dashes of pepper
- 3 dashes of onion powder
- 3 dashes of garlic powder
- 1/3 cup of diced red onions
- 2 avocados sliced and diced
- 1 tomato sliced and diced
- 1 teaspoons of olive oil
- 2 tablespoons of light Italian dressing

Instructions:
- In a large skillet, use the olive oil to sauté shrimp for 4-5 minutes on each side. Season with pepper, onion powder, garlic powder, garlic and herb seasoning while sautéing.
- In a large bowl, combine spinach, onions, avocado and Italian dressing. Mix well.
- Top with sautéed shrimp.

Cauliflower Stir Fry

Total Time: 20 minutes
Prep time: 15 minutes
Cook time: 5 minutes

Yield: 4 servings

Equipment:
Cheese grater or food processor

Ingredients:
- 1 medium-sized head of cauliflower
- 2 tablespoons sesame oil
- 1 small bag of shredded carrots (feel free to shred your own)
- 2 garlic clove, minced
- 1 cup frozen peas
- 2 eggs
- 2 tablespoons low sodium soy sauce
- 1 cup green onions sliced and diced

Instructions:
- Shred cauliflower with cheese grater or by food processor. It should resemble grains of rice.
- Heat 1 tablespoon sesame oil in a large skillet over medium low heat. Add the carrots and garlic and sauté until fragrant (about 5 minutes). Add the cauliflower, peas, and remaining sesame oil to the pan; Sautee quickly to cook the cauliflower to a soft texture.
- Remove the cauliflower once complete.
- Reduce heat and reuse pan from cauliflower to fry eggs. Stir gently, and continuously until the eggs are fully cooked and chopped up.

- Remove eggs and stir into cauliflower mix.
- Stir in remaining low sodium soy sauce and green onions just before serving.
- Enjoy!

Dessert

Pineapple-OO-La-La

Total Time: 10 minutes
Prep time: 5 minutes
Cook time: 5 minutes

Yield: 2 servings

Ingredients:
- 2 cups frozen pineapple chunks
- 1 cup of almond milk
- 1 Teaspoon of honey
- 1 squirt of whip cream – I prefer the 0 calorie less than 1.2 gm sugar Reddi Whip for a little splurge

Instructions:
- Remove frozen pineapples from freezer and let sit for 2-3 minutes.
- Combine the frozen pineapple, milk, and honey in a blender (or food processor) and blend until the mixture has a smooth consistency.
- Transfer the sorbet to serving dish (bowl) and serve immediately.
- If splurging, top sorbet with 1 teaspoon of whip cream.

Abbreviations

1. ASCVD – Arteriosclerotic cardiovascular disease event
2. CAD – Coronary artery disease
3. HDL – High density lipoproteins
4. LDL – Low density lipoproteins
5. NSTEMI – Non-ST elevation myocardial infarction
6. STEMI – ST elevation myocardial infarction
7. TG – Triglycerides

Appendices

	Units	Appointment 1	3-month Check up	6-month Check up
Appointment Catalog				
Cholesterol				
	LDL			
	HDL			
	Triglycerides			
Glucose				
	Fasting			
	Fed			
	A1C%			
Blood Pressure				

My Goals

Last A1C%: _____   Goal A1C%: _____

Fasting: _____   Fed: _____

Blood Sugar Log

Date	Before Breakfast (coffee)	After Breakfast (coffee)	Before lunch	After lunch	Before Dinner	After Dinner
Special Comments						
Special Comments						
Special Comments						
Special Comments						
Special Comments						

My Goals
Systolic: _____   Diastolic: _____

Blood Pressure Log*			
Date	Time	Pressure (Systolic/Diastolic) mmHg	Special Comments

*Things to keep in mind before taking blood pressure
1. Relax for 5 minutes   2. No smoking
3. Keep feet planted flat on the ground

My Goal: _____lbs./kg   Waist _____inches/cm

Weight Log*

Date Sunday-Saturday	Start Weight (lbs./kg)	End Weight (lbs./kg)	Waist Size (inches/cm)	Special Comments (what did you do well this week?)

*Remember weight loss is not a rapid journey. Be patient, optimistic and take this one day at a time
1. Weigh yourself at the same time of day. 2. Weight weekly is not effective for those with reduce or congestive heart failure (you should weight daily)

References

1. World Health Organization. (2016). The top 10 causes of death (Fact sheet No. 310). Retrieved from http://www.who.int/mediacentre/factsheets/fs310/en/
2. Xu JQ, Murphy SL, Kochanek KD, Bastian BA. Deaths: Final data for 2013. National vital statistics reports; vol 64 no 2. Hyattsville, MD: National Center for Health Statistics. 2016.
3. Jacobson, T.A., Ito, M.K., Maki, K.C. et al. National Lipid Association recommendations for patient centered management of dyslipidemia: part 1- executive summary. *J Clin Lipidol*. 2014; 8: 473–488
4. Csordas A, Bernhard D. *The biology behind the atherothrombotic effects of cigarette smoke. Nat Rev Cardiol*. 2013;10:219–230
5. Messner, Barbara, and David Bernhard. "Smoking and Cardiovascular Disease Significance." Smoking and Cardiovascular Disease Significance | Arteriosclerosis, Thrombosis, and Vascular Biology. N.p., 19 Feb. 2014. Web. 11 Oct. 2016.
6. James PA, Oparil S, Carter BL, et al. 2014 Evidence-Based Guideline for the Management of High Blood Pressure in Adults: Report From the Panel Members Appointed to the Eighth Joint National Committee (JNC 8). JAMA. 2014;311(5):507-520. doi:10.1001/jama.2013.284427.
7. American Diabetes Association. Classification and diagnosis of diabetes. In: 2016 Standards of Medical Care in Diabetes. Diabetes Care. 2016;39:S13-22. Accessed at *http://care.diabetesjournals.org/content/39/Supplement_1/S13.full.pdf* on 20 June 2016.
8. Sotos-Prieto M, Bhupathiraju SN, Mattei J, Fung TT, Li Y, Pan A, Willett WC, Rimm EB, Hu FB. *Changes in diet quality scores and risk of cardiovascular disease among US men and women. Circulation. 2015;132:2212–2219. doi: 10.1161/CIRCULATIONAHA.115.017158*

www.ingramcontent.com/pod-product-compliance
Lightning Source LLC
Chambersburg PA
CBHW050844290526
45792CB00002B/517